THE ACID REFLUX BOOK

The Ultimate Guide to Living Comfortably with Acid Reflux

Dr. Colin C. Longenecker

This book is intended to provide information about Acid Reflux. The information is accurate and true to the best of the author's knowledge and is not meant to substitute for professional medical advice or treatment. The publisher and author are not responsible for any adverse effects or consequences resulting from the use of any of the suggestions, or procedures discussed in this book.

TABLE OF CONTENT

INTRODUCTION................................1

CHAPTER ONE 5

Understanding Acid Reflux..................5

CHAPTER TWO 10

Symptoms of Acid Reflux 10

CHAPTER THREE 14

Diagnosing and Treating Acid Reflux.14

CHAPTER FOUR 18

Natural Remedies for Acid Reflux......18

CHAPTER FIVE 26

Avoiding and Managing Acid Reflux..26

CHAPTER SIX 30

Proven Strategies for Controlling Acid

REFLUX 30

CHAPTER SEVEN 34

LIVING WITH ACID REFLUX 34

CONCLUSION 38

INTRODUCTION

Welcome to The Acid Reflux Book! If you are suffering from Acid Reflux, you have come to the right place for relief. This book is designed to help you take control of your health and find natural solutions to your Acid Reflux issues.

This book provides essential information about Acid Reflux and how to treat it, including an overview of what it is and how it affects your body, and how to diagnose, treat, and prevent it. It offers comprehensive guidance on nutrition, lifestyle changes, and natural remedies to help you manage your Acid Reflux symptoms.

Acid Reflux is a common condition, affecting millions of people worldwide. It can be painful and uncomfortable, and it can interfere with everyday life. The good news is that there are ways to manage it and reduce its symptoms. This book provides a comprehensive guide on how to do so.

The book starts with an overview of Acid Reflux and its causes. You will learn the different types of Acid Reflux and its various symptoms. You will also learn about the risk factors and how to identify them.

The next section of the book covers nutrition and lifestyle changes that can help you manage your Acid Reflux. You will learn about which foods to eat and which ones to avoid, as well as how to make healthy lifestyle changes that can reduce your symptoms.

The book then dives into natural remedies for Acid Reflux. You will learn about herbs, supplements, and other natural remedies that can help you reduce your symptoms. You will also learn about alternative therapies, such as yoga and meditation, that can help you find relief.

Finally, the book offers guidance on how to prevent Acid Reflux from coming back. You will learn about lifestyle modifications, such as avoiding certain foods, and how to make changes to your diet and lifestyle that can help you stay healthy.

If you are looking for a comprehensive guide to Acid Reflux, The Acid Reflux Book is the perfect resource. It provides easy-to-understand information on what Acid Reflux is, how to diagnose and treat it, and how to prevent it from coming back. Whether you are looking for natural solutions or lifestyle modifications, this book can help you find relief.

CHAPTER ONE

Understanding Acid Reflux

Do you experience a burning sensation in your chest accompanied by a sour taste in your mouth? You may be suffering from acid reflux. Acid reflux, or gastroesophageal reflux disease (GERD), is a common digestive disorder that affects millions of people worldwide. Unfortunately, most people don't understand the causes and treatments of acid reflux, leading to a lack of effective treatments.

The Acid Reflux Book is an essential resource for those looking to gain a better understanding of acid reflux and how to manage their symptoms. Written by a leading doctor in the field of gastroenterology, this book provides detailed information about the symptoms, causes, and treatments for acid reflux.

The Acid Reflux Book provides readers with a comprehensive understanding of acid reflux. Readers will learn about the anatomy and physiology of the gastrointestinal tract, the causes and symptoms of acid reflux, and the available treatments for this condition. This book also provides clear and concise instructions for lifestyle changes that can help to reduce the symptoms of acid reflux.

The Acid Reflux Book offers readers an extensive list of foods that should be avoided if they suffer from acid reflux. It also provides information on the importance of avoiding certain lifestyle habits, such as smoking and eating late at night, that can worsen the symptoms of acid reflux.

The Acid Reflux Book is an invaluable resource for anyone who wants to gain a better understanding of acid reflux. This book provides readers with the information they need to make informed decisions about their health. With its easy-to-understand language and detailed illustrations, this book is the perfect guide to understanding and managing acid reflux.

If you are looking to gain a better understanding of acid

reflux and how to manage its symptoms, The Acid Reflux Book is the perfect resource. This book provides readers with an in-depth look at the causes, symptoms, and treatments of acid reflux. With its comprehensive information and clear instructions, The Acid Reflux Book is an invaluable resource for anyone looking to take control of their health and reduce the symptoms of acid reflux.

CHAPTER TWO

Symptoms of Acid Reflux

Millions of individuals throughout the world suffer from acid reflux, a common digestive condition. A foul taste in the mouth, a burning sensation in the chest, and pressure or discomfort in the stomach are its defining characteristics. Acid reflux symptoms can be disruptive to daily life and can range from mild to incapacitating. Understanding the symptoms and signs of acid reflux will help you take control of your illness and find the treatment you require.

Heartburn is the most typical sign of acid reflux. A

burning sensation originates in the chest and sometimes travels up the neck. It frequently comes with a sour taste in the mouth and can get worse if you lie down right after eating or eating food. Bloating, belching, nausea, and a sore throat might also be signs.

If acid reflux is left untreated, it might cause more problems. This can include chest pain that may be mistaken for a heart attack, trouble swallowing, and weight loss. Acid reflux may also be associated with chronic coughing, hoarseness, and asthma. Acid reflux can harm the esophagus over time, resulting in ulcers, scarring, and potentially Barrett's esophagus, a precancerous condition.

It's vital to discuss acid reflux with your doctor if you have any of the symptoms. They can aid in making a diagnosis and selecting the most appropriate course of action. Changes in lifestyle, such as abstaining from foods, can help lessen the symptoms. To help regulate the disease, prescription medications may also be used.

The good news is that acid reflux can be successfully treated and managed. Knowing the symptoms and indications of acid reflux might help you spot the problem early and get the necessary therapy. You can receive relief from acid reflux and resume your normal activities with the proper med/lifestyle regimen.

The Acid Reflux Book can be useful if you or someone you know is experiencing acid reflux symptoms. Detailed information on the causes, diagnosis, and treatment of acid reflux is provided in this book. It also provides advice on how to control your symptoms and deal with acid reflux daily. You can take charge of your illness and find the treatment you require with The Acid Reflux Book.

CHAPTER THREE

Diagnosing and Treating Acid Reflux

Acid reflux, also known as GERD (gastroesophageal reflux disease), is a condition in which the contents of the stomach flow back up into the esophagus, causing burning pain, chest tightness, and other unpleasant symptoms. This can be a chronic and debilitating condition, but it is often treatable with lifestyle modifications and medications.

The first step in diagnosing and treating acid reflux is to visit your doctor. Your doctor will perform a physical examination, ask about your symptoms, and review your medical history. Your doctor may recommend laboratory tests or imaging studies to help identify the cause of your acid reflux. The cause of your acid reflux may be something other than GERD.

If you are diagnosed with acid reflux, your doctor may recommend lifestyle modifications to help manage your symptoms. These modifications may include avoiding certain foods, eating smaller meals, avoiding lying down shortly after eating and avoiding eating late at night. Quitting smoking and reducing stress can also help reduce the symptoms of acid reflux.

If lifestyle modifications are not enough to manage your symptoms, your doctor may recommend medications to help reduce the amount of acid produced in your stomach. These medications include proton pump inhibitors (PPIs) and H2 blockers. In some cases, surgery may be recommended to help control the symptoms of acid reflux.

Acid reflux can be a frustrating and painful condition, but it is often treatable with lifestyle changes and medications. If you are experiencing symptoms of acid reflux, make an appointment with your doctor to discuss a treatment plan. With the right combination of lifestyle modifications and medications, you can help keep your acid reflux under control.

Acid reflux should not limit your life. With the right diagnosis and treatment, you can control your symptoms and enjoy life to the fullest. Don't let acid reflux keep you from living your life to the fullest – get the help you need today.

Drinking green juice with ginger is an easy and delicious way to get your daily dose of fruits and vegetables. It's packed with nutrients and flavor, and it can help to protect your body from disease. So, give this powerful juice a try and start enjoying the health benefits of green juice with ginger today!

CHAPTER FOUR

Natural Remedies for Acid Reflux

Millions of individuals all over the world suffer from acid reflux, commonly known as gastroesophageal reflux disease (GERD), which is a common digestive ailment. After eating, there is a burning sensation in the chest, there is a sour taste in the mouth, and food or acid is regurgitated. If left untreated, it can cause major consequences and be a highly uncomfortable, if not painful, condition. Fortunately, numerous natural treatments for acid reflux can offer relief and aid in avoiding additional issues.

A lifestyle change is one of the best natural treatments for acid reflux. The key to reducing symptoms is to eat smaller meals more frequently, avoid items that cause reflux, and avoid lying down right after eating. Maintaining a healthy weight is also crucial because being overweight can put additional strain on the stomach and make acid reflux symptoms worse. Meals should be taken slowly, and drinking alcohol and caffeine in excess should be avoided.

Many natural therapies help relieve acid reflux in addition to lifestyle changes. The use of herbs and spices is one of the most often used natural treatments. Ginger is a popular option because it can calm an upset stomach and reduce motion sickness. Fennel, peppermint, and chamomile are additional plants that can help with acid reflux symptoms.

Make sure to drink plenty of water to avoid acid reflux as another natural treatment. By neutralizing stomach acid, drinking lots of water throughout the day might help lessen the symptoms of acid reflux. Additionally, it's crucial to refrain from consuming too much water with meals as this can raise your risk of acid reflux.

Probiotics can also help treat acid reflux, to finish. Beneficial bacteria known as probiotics support intestinal health. They can aid in easing acid reflux symptoms by reestablishing the proper balance of beneficial bacteria in the gut, which helps facilitate a more efficient digesting process.

These organic treatments for acid reflux might ease the bothersome GERD symptoms and lessen the chance of developing further issues. These natural treatments for acid reflux can be a fantastic place to start, but it's vital to talk to your doctor before trying any new ones. It is possible to locate a natural solution that works for you and provides relief from your symptoms with a little bit of effort and focus.

Nothing beats a combination of lifestyle modifications and natural therapies for acid reflux, in the end. Smaller meals, staying hydrated, avoiding particular food triggers, and utilizing the health benefits of herbs and spices can all help lessen the symptoms of acid reflux. Additionally, including probiotics in your diet can support improved digestive health by re-establishing the balance of healthy bacteria in the stomach. You can get relief from acid reflux symptoms and aid in averting further difficulties by using a mix of these natural treatments and lifestyle modifications.

FOODS TO EAT

Acid reflux is an uncomfortable and often painful condition that many people struggle with. It is caused by a weakened or damaged lower esophageal sphincter, which allows stomach acid to move up the esophagus and causes a burning sensation in the chest and throat. Eating certain foods can trigger the symptoms of acid reflux, but many foods can help reduce the severity of the condition. Here is a list of foods to eat for acid reflux that are both powerful and persuasive:

1. Fruits and Vegetables: Fruits and vegetables are some of the best foods for acid reflux. They are high in fiber, which helps to fill up the stomach and prevent acid reflux symptoms. Fruits like apples, bananas, and melon are great options, as well as vegetables like broccoli, cabbage, and kale.

2. Oatmeal: Oatmeal is a great option for those suffering from acid reflux. It is high in fiber and helps to absorb stomach acid. Plus, it is filling enough to help keep you feeling full throughout the day.

3. Whole Grain Bread: Whole-grain bread is a great option for those with acid reflux. It is high in fiber, which helps to reduce the symptoms of acid reflux. Plus, it is light and easy to digest, which makes it easier on the stomach.

4. Lean Protein: Lean proteins, like fish, chicken, and eggs, are great options for those with acid reflux. They are low in fat and provide the body with important amino

acids. Plus, they are easy to digest, which helps reduce the symptoms of acid reflux.

5. Almond Milk: Almond milk is a great option for those with acid reflux. It is low in fat and high in calcium, which is important for neutralizing stomach acid. Plus, it is a great source of protein, which helps to keep you feeling full.

6. Ginger: Ginger is a great option for those with acid reflux. It is known to help reduce the symptoms of acid reflux. Plus, it is also a great anti-inflammatory and can help reduce the pain associated with acid reflux.

7. Yogurt: A yogurt is a great option for those with acid reflux. It is high in probiotics, which can help to reduce the symptoms of acid reflux. Plus, it is a great source of calcium and protein, which can help to keep you feeling full.

These are just a few of the many powerful and persuasive foods to eat for acid reflux. Eating a balanced diet of fruits, vegetables, lean proteins, and whole grains can help to reduce the symptoms of acid reflux. Plus, avoiding processed foods and eating smaller meals throughout the day, can help to prevent the symptoms of acid reflux from occurring. Eating the right foods can make a big difference in managing acid reflux, so be sure to give these powerful and persuasive foods a try.

FOODS TO AVOID

Acid reflux is a common digestive issue that can cause a variety of unpleasant symptoms ranging from heartburn to chest pain. It is important to be aware of which foods can trigger symptoms and to avoid them to reduce the severity of acid reflux flare-ups. Here are some of the most common foods to avoid if you suffer from acid reflux.

Firstly, it is important to avoid certain beverages if you suffer from acid reflux. These include coffee, tea, and soda, as they are all highly acidic and can cause irritation to the esophagus. Additionally, it is important to avoid alcoholic beverages, as they can relax the esophageal sphincter and allow acid to reflux more easily.

Secondly, certain fried, fatty, and greasy foods are best avoided if you suffer from acid reflux. These types of foods are harder to digest and can linger in the stomach for longer periods, increasing the chances of acid reflux. Additionally, foods that are high in fat can also relax the esophageal sphincter, potentially allowing acid to reflux more easily.

Thirdly, it is important to avoid spicy foods as these can cause irritation to the esophagus and aggravate acid reflux symptoms. Additionally, it is important to avoid acidic foods such as citrus fruits, tomatoes, and tomato-based sauces. These can all irritate the esophagus and cause acid reflux symptoms.

Fourthly, it is also important to avoid certain high-fiber foods such as beans, legumes, and cruciferous vegetables. These can all cause excessive gas and bloating which can aggravate acid reflux symptoms. Furthermore, it is important to avoid processed foods and foods that are high in sugar, as these can irritate the esophagus and trigger acid reflux.

Finally, it is important to avoid eating large meals or eating late at night. Eating large meals can overwhelm the stomach and make it difficult for the stomach to properly digest the food, leading to acid reflux. Additionally, eating late at night can also increase the chances of acid reflux, as lying down after eating can make it easier for acid to reflux.

In conclusion, it is important to be aware of which foods can trigger acid reflux and to avoid them to reduce the severity of symptoms. These include certain beverages, fried, fatty, and greasy foods, spicy foods, acidic foods, high-fiber foods, processed foods, and foods that are high in sugar. Additionally, it is important to avoid eating large meals and eating late at night. Following these tips can help reduce the severity of acid reflux symptoms.

CHAPTER FIVE

Avoiding and Managing Acid Reflux

A medical ailment called acid reflux, commonly referred to as gastroesophageal reflux disease (GERD), occurs when the stomach's contents, including acid and bile, travel back up the esophagus and into the throat. Heartburn, a burning sensation, chest pain, a foul taste in the mouth, and regurgitation can all result from this. There are a few useful techniques to prevent and manage acid reflux, even though it can be an uncomfortable and even painful experience.

Finding out which meals seem to cause acid reflux is

the first step in preventing and treating it. Spicy or acidic foods, fried foods, and foods heavy in fat are typical offenders. It's crucial to keep a meal journal to discover the items that seem to set off your acid reflux. It is possible to lessen the likelihood of suffering acid reflux by avoiding these meals or just consuming them in moderation.

Keeping an eye on your portion sizes is another method to prevent and treat acid reflux. Eating smaller meals frequently throughout the day is crucial since eating too much can cause stomach acid to travel back up the esophagus. To make meals simpler to digest, it's also beneficial to eat slowly and chew each bite thoroughly.

Reducing stress might also lessen the likelihood of developing acid reflux. The amount of stomach acid produced can rise back up the esophagus because of stress. Reduce acid reflux by learning stress-reduction techniques like yoga, deep breathing, or physical activity.

It's also critical to pay attention to your sleeping patterns. It's best to wait at least three hours after eating before lying down because doing so can create acid reflux. Raising the head of your bed a little bit can also assist prevent stomach acid from entering the esophagus.

Finally, if you experience frequent acid reflux, you should talk to your doctor. You can create a unique management strategy for the disease with the assistance of your doctor. This could entail a change in lifestyle, medication, or additional therapies.

These easy steps can help you manage and prevent acid reflux. Acid reflux can be prevented by knowing what foods cause it, limiting your portions, managing your stress, sleeping in the appropriate position, and consulting your doctor. By following these instructions, you can get relief from the unpleasant acid reflux symptoms.

CHAPTER SIX

Proven Strategies for Controlling Acid Reflux

When stomach acid runs back into the esophagus, it causes acid reflux, which results in a burning sensation in the chest and neck. Here are some tried-and-true methods for reducing acid reflux:

Eat smaller, more frequent meals rather than larger ones because large meals might increase acid production in the stomach and aggravate acid reflux symptoms. Smaller, more frequent meals can aid in lowering the production of acid.

Avoid trigger foods: For some people, some foods can

cause symptoms of acid reflux. Spicy and fatty foods, chocolate, coffee, alcohol, and citrus fruits are examples of common trigger foods. Keeping your intake of these items under limits can help you manage acid reflux symptoms.

Lose weight: Being overweight increases the risk of acid reflux by placing pressure on the stomach. The frequency and intensity of symptoms can both be lessened with weight loss.

Raise the head of the bed: By elevating the head as you sleep, you might lessen acid reflux symptoms at night. Use a wedge cushion or put blocks under the legs of the headboard to raise the bed's head.

Eat nothing before going to bed because doing so increases your chance of experiencing acid reflux symptoms at night. It's preferable to wait at least three hours after eating before going to bed.

Quit smoking: Smoking relaxes the muscle that keeps the esophagus from the stomach, which makes acid reflux symptoms worse. Smoking cessation can lessen symptoms and enhance general health.

Control your stress: Stress can make acid reflux symptoms worse. Deep breathing, meditation, and yoga are all effective ways to manage stress and lessen its symptoms.

Think about medication: Medications including antacids, H2 blockers, and proton pump inhibitors can help lessen the amount of acid produced in the stomach if lifestyle adjustments aren't sufficient to control acid reflux symptoms.

If acid reflux symptoms last for a long time or become severe, it's necessary to consult a doctor. They can aid in choosing the most appropriate course of action for any patient's needs.

CHAPTER SEVEN

Living with Acid Reflux

Acid reflux can make daily life difficult, but there are strategies to control your symptoms and lead a happy, healthy life. Gastroesophageal reflux disease, often known as acid reflux, is a disorder where stomach acid leaks into the esophagus and causes a burning feeling in the chest and neck. Heartburn, chest pain, trouble swallowing, and an unpleasant aftertaste are just a few of the symptoms that can range in severity from mild to severe.

Understanding the causes that can cause acid reflux is the first step in managing it. Spicy foods, fatty foods, alcohol, coffee, chocolate, and citrus fruits are typical triggers. Keeping away from certain foods can lessen the symptoms. In addition, consuming fewer, smaller meals more frequently throughout the day rather than three large ones can help lower the level of stomach acid.

Maintaining a healthy body weight is also crucial. Increased strain on the stomach from being overweight might cause more acid to reflux into the esophagus. Exercise can enhance digestion and aid in weight loss. Additionally crucial are eating gently and limiting one's intake.

Acid reflux is frequently treated with prescription medications. Antacids can lessen symptoms by neutralizing gastric acid. Proton pump inhibitors can lessen the quantity of stomach acid produced. The optimal drugs for you can only be determined by talking to your doctor.

Making lifestyle adjustments can also aid in symptom reduction. Acid reflux can be lessened and stomach acid production can be decreased by quitting smoking. Additionally, wearing loose-fitting clothing can ease the strain on the stomach. Avoiding lying down just after eating can keep stomach acid under control.

Although managing acid reflux can be challenging, there are things you can do to lessen your symptoms and enhance your general quality of life. Acid reflux can be lessened by avoiding trigger foods, maintaining a healthy weight, and changing one's lifestyle. Taking prescription drugs as directed can also aid with symptom management. Living with acid reflux can be handled with the proper care and control.

CONCLUSION

Acid reflux is a common but serious condition that can have a significant impact on your life. It can cause heartburn, chest pain, regurgitation, difficulty swallowing, coughing, and other unpleasant symptoms. In some cases, it can even lead to more serious complications such as esophageal cancer.

Fortunately, there are several ways to manage and treat acid reflux. Diet and lifestyle changes, medications, and lifestyle remedies can all help to reduce the symptoms and the frequency of acid reflux. Eating smaller meals and avoiding certain trigger foods, avoiding lying down after eating, and not smoking or drinking alcohol can all help to reduce your symptoms.

Medications, such as antacids, proton pump inhibitors,

and H2 blockers, can also be used to manage acid reflux. These medications can help to reduce the amount of acid produced in the stomach, reduce the amount of time acid stays in the stomach, and reduce the chance of the acid refluxing into the esophagus.

Finally, lifestyle remedies such as yoga, meditation, and lifestyle changes can also help to reduce the symptoms of acid reflux. These remedies can help to reduce stress and anxiety, which can be a major factor in acid reflux. In addition, lifestyle changes such as avoiding caffeine and alcohol, not eating late at night, and avoiding tight clothing can also help to reduce symptoms.

Overall, acid reflux is a serious condition that can have a significant impact on your life. Fortunately, there are a variety of treatments and lifestyle changes that can help to reduce the symptoms and frequency of acid reflux. With the right diet and lifestyle changes, medications, and lifestyle remedies, you can manage your acid reflux and live a happier, healthier life.

So, if you are suffering from acid reflux, don't delay. Take the necessary steps to manage your condition and take back control of your life. With the right diet and lifestyle changes, medications, and lifestyle remedies, you can live a life free from the symptoms of acid reflux.

www.ingramcontent.com/pod-product-compliance
Lightning Source LLC
Chambersburg PA
CBHW071118220526
45467CB00004B/1944
* 9 7 9 8 3 8 8 5 6 3 8 7 3 *